'This really is a great book. Richard Bertschinger achieves a brightness and levity in the pages of this volume that reflects his teaching – a lightness of being that is both mischievous and benevolent, and authentically Taoist. In retaining the mythic poetry through which Taoists describe human experience and the wider macrocosm (the purple dragon of the tongue, the heavenly column of the neck), Richard remains true to the transformative language of this treasured tradition that seeks, in his words, to make anew our experience each day.'

– *Paul Hougham, author of* The Atlas of Mind, Body and Spirit, *past Principal of The College of Traditional Acupuncture, UK*

'*Everyday Qigong Practice* is an excellent introduction for anyone wishing to improve their health and wellbeing. The book presents simply and in a conducive spirit the essence of this empirical art, invented and developed in China. Included are a selection of traditional and widely practiced Qigong exercise systems, that will hopefully inspire many people to find a recommended and qualified teacher of traditional Qigong where they live and safely further their daily practice.

I can personally attest to the practicality and beauty of these regimens, that if practised on a regular basis over time will certainly enrich one's physical, mental and emotional being.'

– *Sifu Gary Wragg, Chief Instructor and Director of Wu's Tai Chi Chuan Academy London, UK and Europe, Founder Member and Former Chairman of the Tai Chi Union for Great Britain*

'I have studied Qigong with Richard for more than twenty years. His approach to teaching is so simple and clear it's easy to think you've discovered the exercise yourself. Yet every session reveals depths. I would recommend him to everyone.'

– *Russell, Qigong student*

T0299602

'Richard has managed to condense some very ancient wisdom into these pages, which I found very readable and easy to follow. If these exercises are followed, the "Energy of Life" will flow and be enhanced, contributing to a healthier body and mind. I enjoyed the beautiful Chinese drawings and the poems in the book that help to make it so appealing.'

– Dr Phil Jackson, retired GP

'I have always found any form difficult to follow and so for some time I ignored Richard's invitation to attend his Qigong class. However, Richard has proven himself to be subtly persuasive and, having "psyched myself up", I found myself in his class one January morning. I soon found Richard's approach gentle and non-regimental and also found that there is room for fun and lightness of self. My fear and embarrassment dissipated and now I enjoy my practice. I enjoy being at one with myself, whether practising in the studio or at home. In the eighteen months since I first began Qigong I have found my confidence and overall wellbeing has improved greatly.'

– Wendy, Qigong student

EVERYDAY QIGONG PRACTICE

by the same author

The Secret of Everlasting Life
The First Translation of the Ancient Chinese Text on Immortality
Richard Bertschinger
ISBN 978 1 84819 048 1
eISBN 978 0 85701 054 4

Yijing, Shamanic Oracle of China
A New Book of Change
Translated with commentary by Richard Bertschinger
ISBN 978 1 84819 083 2
eISBN 978 0 85701 066 7

of related interest

Chinese Shamanic Cosmic Orbit Qigong
Esoteric Talismans, Mantras, and Mudras
in Healing and Inner Cultivation
Master Zhongxian Wu
ISBN 978 1 84819 056 6
eISBN 978 0 85701 059 9

Fire Dragon Meridian Qigong
Essential NeiGong for Health and Spiritual Transformation
Master Zhongxian Wu and Dr Karin Taylor Wu
ISBN 978 1 84819 103 7
eISBN 978 0 85701 085 8

Seeking the Spirit of The Book of Change
8 Days to Mastering a Shamanic Yijing
(I Ching) Prediction System
Master Zhongxian Wu
ISBN 978 1 84819 020 7
eISBN 978 0 85701 007 0

EVERYDAY
Qigong
PRACTICE

—— RICHARD BERTSCHINGER ——

Illustrated by Harriet E. J. Lewars

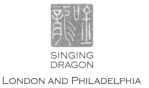

SINGING
DRAGON

LONDON AND PHILADELPHIA

Disclaimer: No health claims are made in this book. If in doubt or in pain consult your physician. Unusual lumps or bumps should not be massaged – go and get them checked!

First published in 2013
by Singing Dragon
an imprint of Jessica Kingsley Publishers
116 Pentonville Road
London N1 9JB, UK
and
400 Market Street, Suite 400
Philadelphia, PA 19106, USA

www.singingdragon.com

Copyright © Richard Bertschinger 2013
Illustrations copyright © Harriet E. J. Lewars 2013

Library of Congress Cataloging in Publication Data
A CIP catalog record for this book is available from the Library of Congress

British Library Cataloguing in Publication Data
A CIP catalogue record for this book is available from the British Library

ISBN 978 1 84819 117 4
eISBN 978 0 85701 097 1

Printed and bound in Great Britain

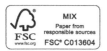

This small book summarizes a few of the exercises I have taught over the past twenty-five years in my Qigong classes. Sources are traditional, and were adjusted to the class. I also need to acknowledge my instruction at Chengdu College of Chinese Medicine in 1986. My pupils have led the way, as ever. Indeed to all of them I'm eternally grateful. My teacher Gia-fu Feng (d. 1985) used to say 'every blade of grass in its right place'. To him also I owe an inestimable debt. On the wall of the bath chamber of Emperor Tang (founder of the Shang dynasty in 1766 BCE) was inscribed, in gold letters: *as the sun makes it anew, day by day make it new, every day make it anew.* This is the practice of Qigong.

Introduction

There are three things this book aims to teach: regulation of the body, regulation of the breathing and regulation of the mind. This is the 'triple harmony' which lies at the heart of Qigong practice.

These exercises are extensively documented, at least back to Han dynasty times (c. 200 BCE) when the like were depicted on the walls of the Mawangdui tombs, as well as being ridiculed in the *Zhuangzi* book as 'bear hangings' or 'bird-neck twistings'.

First come three short poems giving some instruction in *Early Morning Meditation*, or waking exercises of the Taoists. They concentrate on swallowing saliva, twisting joints, and rubbing, patting and pressing the body to mobilize the qi, blood and fluids. Their energies are then consolidated in the belly.

Next comes the ever-popular *An Eight-Sectioned Brocade* (Baduan Jin), popular in Taoist circles in the West. Following this the contemporary *Three Circles Posture*, which I learnt in China in 1986, also known as the Standing Pole and Holding the Ball, among other names.

My Chinese teacher said: 'Nothing seems to be going on, but we know plenty is going on!' The Three Circles is a *dynamic* meditation, inhibiting the cerebral activity of the brain through activating sympathetic and parasympathetic auto-regulation, a real gem.

Interestingly enough, the character Tiao 調 ('regulation') in classical Chinese means also 'to tune up', 'to mix together' or 'to mash', as in the Yorkshire expression 'to mash tea'. So it can be seen that rules in Traditional Chinese Medicine are descriptive, as well as prescriptive. There is no rigid divide, which also illustrates the underlying principle of Yin and Yang – two forces which are at once in opposition, at once complementary.

During your practice of these simple exercises there may well be a need for personal dialogue. The mind is often asking questions and seeking solutions. Do not be too self-critical. The genius of the Chinese approach is to begin with the body, and instruct it carefully. Then the breathing becomes self-regulatory and the cultivation of the mind occurs naturally. In Chinese this is called 'self-so' or 'self-suchness' – Ziran 自然; also translated as 'spontaneity'.

Other forms of meditation (which occupy the 'middle-zone' of the mind, and do not begin with the body) may risk muddying the water with their constant danger of self-aggrandisement. The relaxation of the muscles must come first.

This is followed by *Ten Aggrievement Exercises*. These are good for early morning loosening and combating that 'grumpy' mood that comes on so easily with age. Keep the mind bright and forward-looking as you practise – mix and match, and 'make it up somewhat' as you go along; these exercises are creative. Their aim is to move qi. A modicum of over-exertion might be essayed. But take care.

Then come *The Three Lowerings*, an exercise for sound sleep. This is a subtle and gentle method of encouraging the self-regulation of the autonomic response, the 'rest and digest' reflex. Cultivating quiet is an art with a long Taoist tradition; and peaceful sleep a Taoist art. You may combine this exercise with the rubbing which follows. Rubbing is self-explanatory. Suffice it to say, self-massage and rubbing can be practised even when you are sick, or convalescing. Indeed, at this time they are *especially* indicated.

Lastly I include some brief extracts from the old Taoist texts. They describe the more esoteric side of Qigong, but it all begins and ends in daily practice.

Select one of the following exercises and follow it through diligently. Personal instruction is best and you should try to find a teacher in your local area. For the Brocades, or morning waking exercises, a hundred days of practice of 10–20 minutes could be tried. You may miss the odd day. But if you are convalescing, you can practise three or four times a day. At the same time, restrict your diet, sexual activity and over-work for best results. These exercises can also be carried around and fitted into a busy schedule. No apparatus or special court is required! They are suitable for young or old, the well or infirm, although they have a special relevance for those recovering from illness. The preface to my Chinese copy of the works of the Taoist scholar and poet Zhuangzi ends with a summary of what can be gained through human effort:

> *Past and present hearts differ, yet the hearts of the past and present peoples are the same. We who live in the present, and study the works of old, must use our present hearts to move backward and penetrate the hearts of old. Then heart to heart we will join. How then will there be any ideas to confound us?*

So work hard! The physician Sun Simiao said: 'Cultivating health? It is nothing more than sunlight and water!'

Please write or email if you wish via www.mytaoworld.com.

Early Morning Meditation

These rubbings, pattings and pressings, simple stretches for the limbs, teeth-chomping and shaking are surprisingly effective at presenting oneself to the world. Do not use too much effort at first. Stick to the order and schedule and you will soon develop a routine. If you don't understand a particular line, then omit it.

Some general pointers

Make sure the hands, wrists and shoulders are all relaxed making the moves. Chomping the jaws, allow the whole mouth, cheeks and jaw to be loose. To dry wash the face, stroke gently, using the finger-tips. When you grasp the hair and pull, it strengthens the roots. All this mobilizes blood and qi. Pay special attention to the pauses ('rest awhile'). They allow natural consolidation.

When the 'purple dragon stirs' slowly run the tongue (purple dragon) around between the gums and teeth, the upper and lower jaws. This promotes excellent oral hygiene. The 'neck agenda' is simply a term for that tension often associated with the liver-yang of Chinese medicine.

When you 'pound with loosened fists' always keep the fists and wrists loose, not bunched up tight. This practice is supremely effective in moving blood and qi.

UPON AWAKENING SIT UPRIGHT

close the eyes and dim the mind
hold it fast and still the spirit

chomp the jaws, thirty-six times
dry wash the face, pull down the hands
slowly, firmly, press and pull the face,
half a dozen times

draw the hands back over the scalp
fingers pressing firmly, two or three times
pull the back of the neck,
grasp the hair, and gently pull
slightly sway the heavenly column*

purple dragon** stirs in the teeth,
run the tongue round the gums
upper and lower
left and right

three times one way
three times another,

---

*   neck
**   tongue

gather the fluid and swallow it down
in two or three mouthfuls

imagine it falling, sinking down
sinking to the lower belly

finish with one breath
hold fast the mind and strengthen the spirit

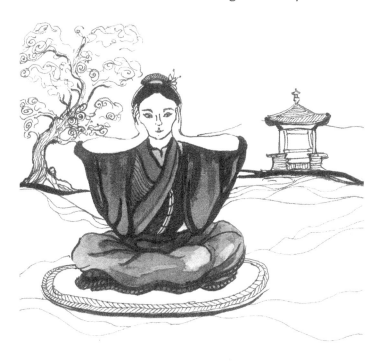

LINK FINGERS AND PRESS ABOVE

stretching the sinews
supporting the sky

let the breath fill the upper chest
lower the hands, then rest awhile

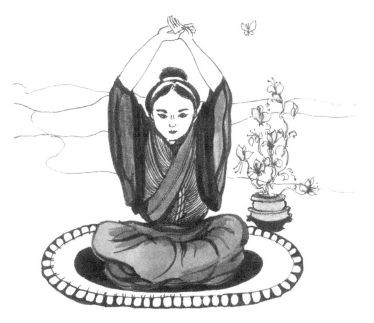

shake hands, rub palms until warm
hold the kidneys' palace, press
as if adorning the back, treasure

rub again and shake the fingers
rub the sides, pinch the waist
thumbs afore, thumbs behind,
deeply take a breath

lift one shoulder, and rotate it
back, down, forward and back up
turn the shoulder hubs
separately and together,
together and apart
four times nine, thirty-six times

turn the neck, place the hands behind,
and rub and press the neck agenda
rub, pull, press, finger and thumb
pressing, kneading

slightly sway the heavenly column
sit upright, rest awhile

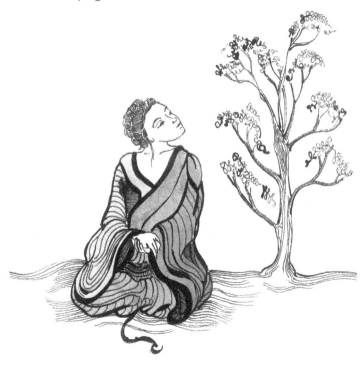

LET THE LEGS LOOSE AND STRETCH

wiggle toes, point them down
turn inwards and out

pull up the big toe, stretch the calf
lower and pat the knees

take the hands and warm them
circle the knees, thirty-six times
round in circles,
round and back again

pat hands again
pinch and pound, with loosened fists
pound thighs, lower belly
loosen everything

loosen fingers, slap forward and back
thighs, belly, groin, back and sides
nurture the warmth
rest awhile

gather the fluid and swallow down
in two or three mouthfuls,
warm hands, warm heart
smile,
think no twisted thoughts*
rest awhile

---

*   a phrase from the Confucian Analects

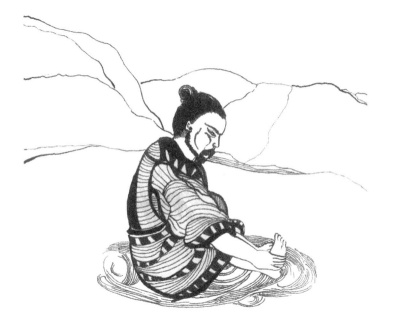

An Eight-Sectioned Brocade

The graceful set of exercises which follows has a history that stretches back beyond the Chinese middle ages. They are recorded in sixth-century texts and have enjoyed great popularity on account of their simplicity.

They comprise a single unit, akin to a richly embroidered silken brocade material, in eight sections.

Relax yourself, both physically and mentally, when practising. This is a most important aspect. Use and acknowledge strength, but not force. Repeat each exercise three or four times.

Practise every day, checking your own ability, with a light spirit. Let the breath move freely and naturally throughout. Allow no morbid thoughts.

- Press Up the Sky, Rest Awhile
- Draw the Bow, Both Sides
- Open Ribcage, Left and Right
- Turn Head, Looking Behind
- Punching Fists, Loosely
- Sway Waist, Looking Behind
- Bending Down, Waterfall
- On Toes, Rise and Fall, Rest

PRESS UP THE SKY, REST AWHILE

Raise hands with palms facing upwards, in front of the body. Turn as they pass the chest, to above the head, palms upward. Prop the sky. The heels may be possibly lifted, possibly not. Bring the hands down the way they came. Do not hurry.

This helps the upper chest, relieves fatigue, extends muscles and sinews, relaxes the shoulders and neck; it corrects a slump. It also prepares for the following moves.

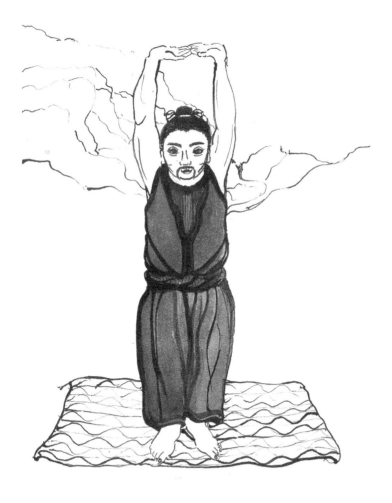

DRAW THE BOW, BOTH SIDES

Take a side-step into the horse-riding posture. Knees bent, as if astride, slightly direct them outward. Do not go too low. Adjust to your own strength. Cross hands alternately and draw out the bow. One arm holds the bow, the other pulling back the string. The fingers of one hand are the arrow; the others draw back steadily the string. You may sweat, but do not get out of breath. Keep shoulders loose.

This exercise improves the breathing, and loosens and treats disorders of the upper limbs. It strengthens the waist, arms, legs and back, and adjusts mind and spirit.

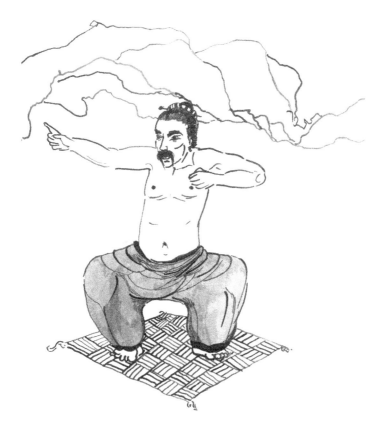

OPEN RIBCAGE, LEFT AND RIGHT

Hold palms lightly in front of abdomen. Feet should be shoulder width. Allow hands, fingers and wrists to be quite relaxed. Raise a single hand, palm slanting up, while the other turns and falls. The one above the head; the other near the hip. The opposing knee can also be raised high to strengthen the effect. Return the way you came. Repeat on other side.

This exercise, slowly performed, helps regulate the liver and digestion, and moves flatulence. It helps all rib and side problems and benefits the emotions.

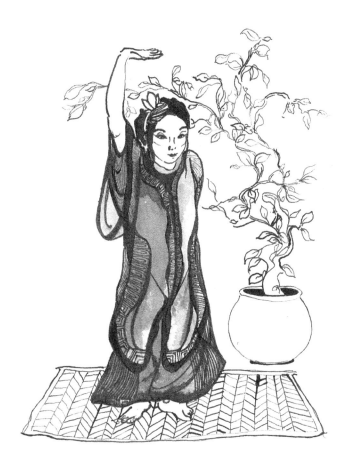

TURN HEAD, LOOKING BEHIND

The backs of the hands press against the small of the back, resting over the kidneys' palace. Else you can leave them loose at the sides. Turn gradually to look backwards, moving the whole body, keeping the feet planted. Turn easily. Return the way you came. Then repeat easily the other side. Move smoothly and gently; do not hold an extreme position.

This movement stimulates the blood around the whole spine. It nourishes the brain, and eliminates tiredness when performed properly. It improves mental hygiene.

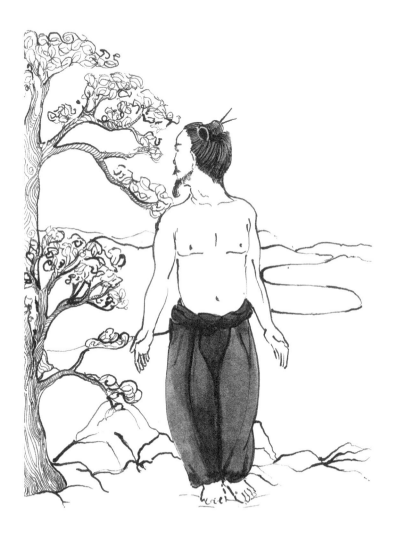

PUNCHING FISTS, LOOSELY

Again in the horse-riding posture, as before, punch fists alternately left and right, diagonally across the body. One fist stretches out rotating in, as the other withdraws, rotating out, pulled back under the armpit. Use some force, with staring eyes. Look forward. Repeat several times. Quick movements are allowed.

This exercise stimulates the cerebral cortex and autonomic system. It promotes circulation and may eliminate 'liver-fire'.

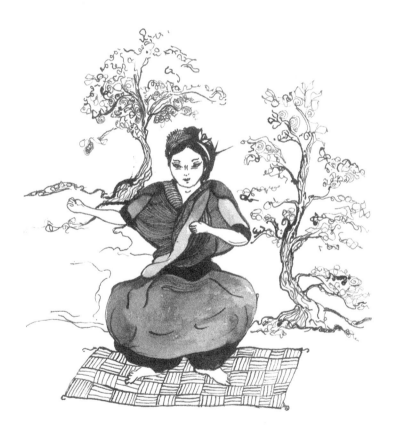

SWAY WAIST, LOOKING BEHIND

In horse-riding posture again, allow palms to rest on thighs, fingers or thumbs inside. Lower the head and bend trunk forward, then sway upper body left while hips are directed to the right. Left arm straightens, right arm bends. Breathe naturally. Return to middle and repeat the other side. You can also turn head behind, with a fierce grimace. The Chinese say this is 'scaring away the demons walking behind you'.

This exercise removes the strain on the nervous system by activating the lower section of the body. It eliminates 'heart-fire', a medical condition which is not easily removed by rest. It also strengthens the waist.

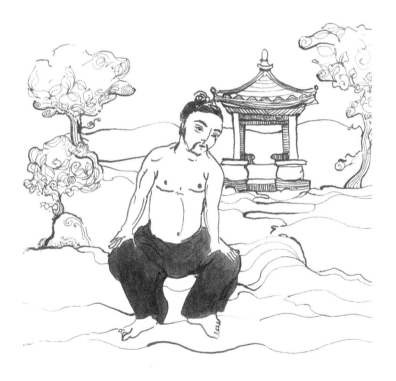

BENDING DOWN, WATERFALL

Feet must be a natural width apart. Bend forward to reach down towards the toe tips. Reach down as far as is comfortable and a little more. Upper body falls down, then hands and arms sweep up again, palms up to chest. And repeat. Imagine the passage of water. Simulate a water-wheel or waterfall. Knees should not be locked. Breathe naturally. Go slowly.

You should not perform this exercise if you have uncontrolled blood-pressure. It strengthens the lumbar region, and prevents and eases back-ache. It improves hormonal function.

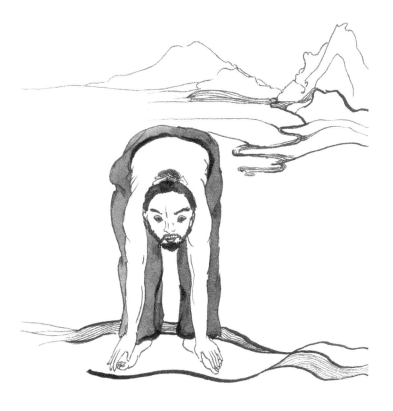

ON TOES, RISE AND FALL, REST

Feet together, slowly let the heels rise and fall together. Palms should be pressed at the sides or, as before, into the small of the back. You may repeat this exercise many times, up to one hundred. This simple form relaxes and brings to a close the Eight-Sectioned Brocade.

The whole Brocade need only be performed through once. But if wished it can be repeated two or three times.

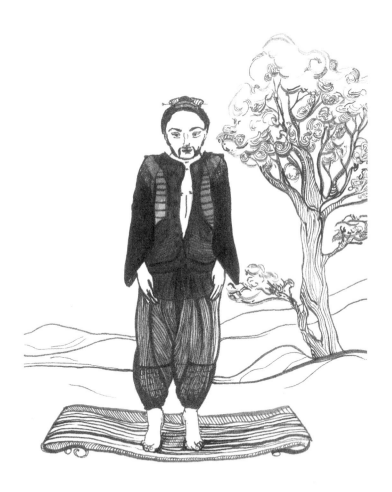

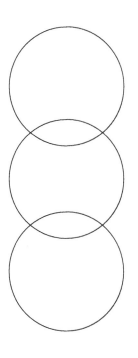

The Three Circles Posture

'When the Tree withers, the leaves fall...
What can we say then?
The Trunk is still visible, a golden wind...'

THE THREE CIRCLES POSTURE is an exercise from contemporary China. I learnt it during my studies at Chengdu College of Chinese Medicine, from the esteemed Doctor Li. It is one of the easiest forms of Qigong to learn, although its practice takes dedication and some skill. However, it is a highly adaptable form of mental and physical education; it is superlative at smoothing and easing the body, the breath and mental condition.

Its particular feature is the conscious relaxation of tension, especially that in the chest and abdomen. Properly performed it results in very little oxygen debt to the muscles; although the pulse rate may slightly increase, respiration is unrestricted. There are no sudden moves or undue stretching. Blood circulation is enhanced and this makes it suitable for those with cardiovascular troubles or the frail. At the same time its crowning achievement is the spontaneous inhibition of the activity of the cerebral cortex. In other words, you may find a world beyond thought – most useful in a cluttered world!

The 'golden wind' mentioned in the poem above is a reference to Taoist alchemy: the gold resides unchanging in the breath of the lungs – the wind, or movement, springing forth, is brought about by the liver.

Stand upright in a quiet location. If you are not up to standing, then practise seated. Choose whatever is appropriate. Prepare yourself beforehand by toileting and making sure you are suitably dressed and warm. Select a place with pleasant associations. A place of work or bedroom is not ideal.

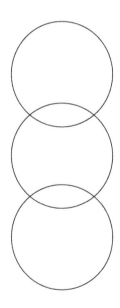

There are three parts to the posture and they progress in this order:

- regulating the body

- regulating the breath

- regulating the mind

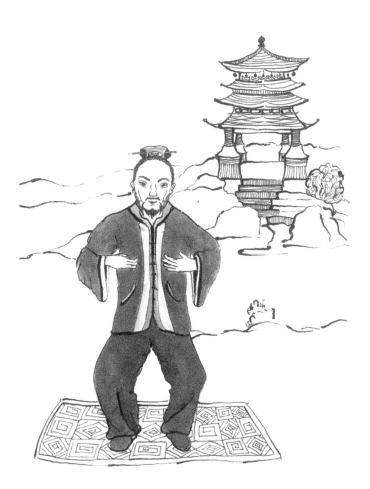

REGULATING THE BODY

Stand upright comfortably with the feet shoulder width apart, and fairly parallel. The arms and hands should be loosely held in front of the lower abdomen, as if embracing a circle. There is another circle between your feet and another between your hands. These are the Three Circles. The head should be held upright, the gaze settled on the horizon. Eyes can be closed, but this is not essential. If thoughts are a problem or you find yourself swaying, then slightly open them.

There are eighteen pointers to this posture and they should be learnt by rote:

1. Feet flat
2. Knees bent and crooked
3. Thighs relaxed
4. Pelvis open
5. Waist fallen
6. Back extended
7. Chest collapsed
8. A line joining stomach...
9. ...and anus
10. Hollow under the arms

11. Elbows dropped

12. Wrists drooped

13. Fingers loose

14. Head suspended

15. Chin pulled in

16. Mouth closed

17. Eyes nearly closed

18. Tongue on roof of mouth

These are the eighteen pointers. They comprise *four lower* (feet, knees, thighs, pelvis), *five lower* (waist, back, chest, stomach, anus), *four upper* (underarms, elbows, wrists, fingers) and *five upper* (head, chin, mouth, eyes, tongue).

When you have held this posture for a comfortable length of time you may close – by drawing the hands back to the lower belly, and closing in the feet. Then stand a while before resuming normal activities. This is the whole of the exercise.

The three essentials

There were three essentials taught at the Chinese college in Sichuan: in performing each posture strive to be *at ease, comfortable* and *natural.*

The above cannot be emphasized enough. There is no merit whatsoever in being competitive in practice. However, striving to be natural is something of an oxymoron!

Stand only as long as you want. It may be two minutes or twenty minutes. This is the fundamental point. Never force it.

Once the posture is comfortable and can be held for a few minutes, you may begin to regulate and quieten the breath.

REGULATING THE BREATH

First it should be said that the process of regulating the breath should not be hurried. It will sometimes, and increasingly often, come about easily, of its own accord. Regulating the body must always come first. Then the essentials of the breath can be attended to. The breath should, at all times, be:

- natural – leave it alone

- not interfered with

- watched simply

Thus the merit in harmonizing the breathing is that it happens very much 'of itself'; it softens almost spontaneously. This is akin to the self-nature of the Buddhists.

This may happen immediately, but it can also take some time. Generally, the practice of the breath builds up after a few weeks' practice. The breath and the attitude of mind are intimately linked.

The Five Words of Breath are *long, deep, slow, even* and *fine*. It should be *as gentle as if drawing on a silken thread*.

Generally encourage the breath to lengthen; it will then naturally deepen and slow down. Then it will become even and fine.

However, the cultivation of the breath is a subtle art, which demands discipline and time.

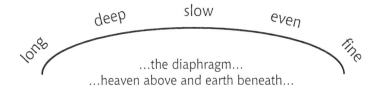

REGULATING THE MIND

Regulating the mind will come of its own accord, as the breath is mastered. But a simple technique to aid you is the counting of the in-breaths and out-breaths. Tie the mind to the breathing and count one to nine (one to six for females). If you lose count then gently bring the mind back and back again, in order to begin the count anew. Do not get frustrated.

Possible problems

As a mnemonic, remember the word BUD: Breathing, Unruly thoughts and Don't. These stand for three common errors made by students of the Three Circles Posture. They are:

- difficulty with the breathing

- difficulty with unruly thoughts

- difficulty generally with any aspect of it, or indeed the whole exercise

The remedy for the first problem is simple. If you have difficulty with the breathing, just remember the three essentials. Remain *at ease*, *comfortable* and *natural* in your behaviour. Don't interfere with the breath. Simply watch it, and leave it alone.

The remedy for unruly thoughts is much the same. Turn your attention to the breath and allow it to flow in and out of its own accord. The thoughts will eventually subside.

The remedy for the third difficulty is also simple. Most probably you have practised enough today and actually don't want to continue the exercise. The time or place may also be inappropriate.

It can be quite likely that you are tired and not recognizing it. Give it up and practise another day.

Good luck. A hundred days of this and you should be flying!

Common hazards

Sometimes the body will tremble or slightly shake, feelings of hot or cold may occur, or there may be slight pains or aches in various parts of the body. These should be accepted as natural movements of the qi or vital energy. They are generally good signs. Try to move the pain around, to another place. But if the pain is too great, then slightly adjust the posture. If the mind becomes possessed of strong thoughts or emotions then finish the posture and do some other mundane tasks, such as washing, sweeping, gardening or domestic duties. You may begin again at another time of the day. It takes a while to find the place and position that suits you.

Keep in mind that there are many contradictions in this posture. Pain or no pain? Tension or relaxation? Focus or non-focus? This is all quite natural. We are still, but also there is movement. Sometimes we feel pain – then it goes. Our muscles will naturally tense and then slacken. The mind does much the same, of its own accord. Just let it be. Good luck!

Ten Aggrievement Exercises

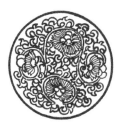

Try a selection or all of these exercises for a week or so. They are purposely constructed to allow some individual expression. Leave the breath alone. Look on them as simple daily stretches. Just a few weeks' daily practice will usually align body and mind. Allow some individual interpretation.

STAND IN A QUIET PLACE

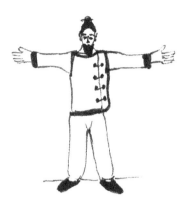

take a deep breath, arms outstretched,
wrists and elbows loose
stand on tip-toe, if you wish
hold a moment, a little longer
and then release,
come back to standing quietly

1 RAISE ARMS TO SHOULDER HEIGHT

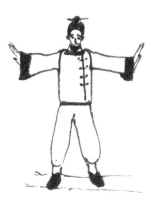

elbows loose, bent, wrists loose, bent
and press sideways, shoulder height
keeping wrists slightly bent, fingers to the sky
act as if *pressing* out

feet may be shoulder width apart, parallel
or toes slightly pointed in

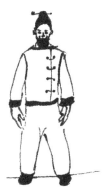

relax, and drop arms and hands back down –
repeat as you wish

2 NOW RAISE ARMS AGAIN AND PRESS

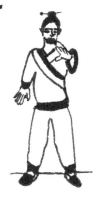

this time, also at shoulder height,
push one arm forward, and one arm
behind
turning the body slightly –
the knees can be slightly unlocked

relax, drop arms back all the way down,
then repeat, on the opposite side
one arm forward, and one arm behind
most importantly, each time unlock the knees

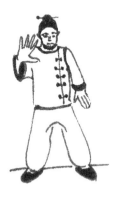

press as if pressing out walls
as if widening, pushing
there's no need to use great effort
some days be dynamic
some days be gentle and gracious
then relax, and arms down

3 LIFT ARMS TO CHEST HEIGHT

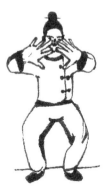

palms up, close to body –
rotate forearms and press palms forward
at the same time, bend knees and squat gently,
go down as far as comfortable, heels down
it is most important you *don't* lean forward
it is better you sink your weight
sink your weight down
the knees should point over the toes
rest, stretch

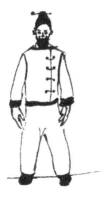

then come back up, and relax –
in this practice, take your time
judge your strength accordingly
act smoothly –
then rest awhile

4 STANDING SIMPLY, RELAXED AND CALM

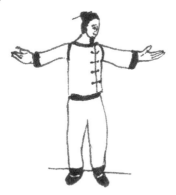

let a little smile flit across your face –
as if you had secret thoughts

as if you knew a secret,
feet shoulder width
raise arms gently to sides
palms up, hands and fingers extended
turn the head, one way and another if you wish
bring the arms down

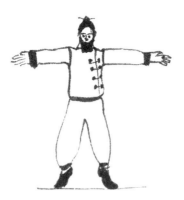

repeat the twisting
turning your body to the right
repeat the turning
twisting your body to the left
palms should be flat and flexible
stretched out as if supporting bowls of water
as if holding a saucer of milk on your palm –
go gently

some days, the knees will bend
some days the knees are reluctant to –

pause:

feel the earth, stand sound, stand solid
lift your toes, then grip the ground –
flex ankles, bend knees
clench fists, be at ease

twist the body, turn and groan
frown and chomp your teeth
clamp the jaws, swallow saliva
breathe *deeply* the stuff of life –

continue:

5 NOW STAND AWHILE

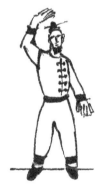

raise one arm, palm facing the sky
close to the body, chest height,
then rotate the forearm, press to the sky
above the head, palm pressing upward
the other arm, stretched down by the side
relax, standing upright –

then repeat on the other side,
practise many times

6 DRAGON ARMS, LEFT AND RIGHT

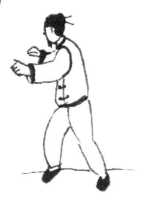

bend knees, twist body, stay upright
eyes fiercely scan behind, prowl

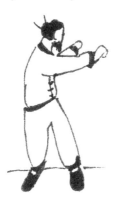

both palms upwards
one ahead, one behind

arms swing left and right
as if imitating the black dragon

7 PROP UP THE SKY

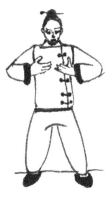

both hands lifting
palms facing up;
flip over palms
push to the heavens
stretch arms alternately

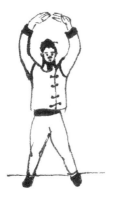

left and right –
let the breath run true

8 TOUCH THE EARTH, LEFT AND RIGHT

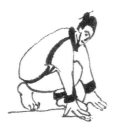

bending the body down
afore and behind
turning the body, left and right
twisting the neck
then

begin the gentle walk...
walking is best wandering
wondering

finish the walk: close

9 STANDING CIRCLES, LARGE ONES

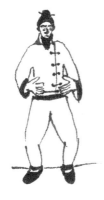

standing circles, small ones
hold the posture
the feet shoulder width apart, or slightly more

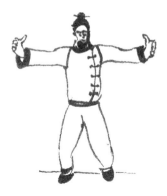

round out the pelvis
round out the chest

10 CLOSE

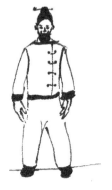

curl, uncurl the back
ripple silently, quietly, settling
feel the flow of the qi

standing – close – be at peace

The Three Lowerings

The Three Lowerings is a standing posture for encouraging quiet and sound sleep. It uses very small movements of the muscles, coordinated with the *outbreath*, in order to redirect blood flow and decrease cortical activity. This also synchronises the sympathetic-parasympathetic system. The trick is in following the gentle breath – without interfering.

> Stand quietly and upright. Feet should be shoulder-width apart, or thereabouts. Eyes are relaxed, half-closed. Allow your hands to rest, palms on the lower belly, below the navel.

> Watch the breathing. On the out-breath, bend the knees slightly, no more than the knees just resting above the end of the toes.

> With the knees slightly bent, allow the breath to enter in slowly, gradually.

On the next breath out, raise the body as you are breathing out, by slightly straightening the knees, back to the original position.

Allow the breath to settle, for a few moments.

Then repeat – no more than three to four times in all.

You may practise again later in the day.

To enhance the effect you may also use the tongue, placing it on the lower palate when you lower the body and bend the knees and on the upper palate when you raise the body and unflex the knees.

You move always on the out-breath.

Try always to breathe through the nose, or at least in through the nose and out through the mouth.

This was an exercise I learnt some years ago for attaining and maintaining sound sleep. It is best practised in the evening before you go to bed. It may also be performed in the morning.

The essence is to approach the posture in the correct frame of mind; quietly and calmly is ideal. Find a pleasant place to stand, with friendly associations. Lower and raise the body with the breath a few times, no more than three or four times in all. *In between each lowering and raising, let the breath settle of its own accord.* This is a most important feature. It is during these few moments that a recovery of the natural cortical activity of the brain is taking place. It embraces the Taoist concept of non-action or *wu-wei*.

Above all it is important to proceed regularly over ten to fourteen days, in a gradual matter. Try to pick around the same time of day. Then you can perhaps take a break.

VARIATION

A variation of this exercise can also be used as a general strengthener for the body, legs and back. In this case make a slow count of five as you lower; make a count of ten as you remain down; and then make a count of fifteen as you come slowly back up. In this case the breath should be allowed to move in and out freely. Again practise only three or four times, in a single session. However, you can put in half a dozen sessions in the day if you wish. This of course increases the stimulating effect.

The Genius of Rubbing

One of the simplest and most effective practices to come out of traditional China is that of rubbing. Rubbing can be practised at any time. But it is best when you are alone and quiet, and can practise regular strokes, presses or just stroking and resting the hands over the area.

It may be divided into rubbing the belly, rubbing the arms, rubbing the knees, rubbing the back, rubbing the face, rubbing the hands and rubbing the feet – but really, heck, you can rub anywhere!

The essentials are to be *gentle* and *even* with your hand movements, and watch how the body responds. Practise regularly two or three times a day to begin with – and then after ten days or so, take a break. Always use a *soft* hand. You will get a better result by pressing *less*, not more, usually. Obviously if you have any lumps, bumps or sores, avoid them.

If your hands are cold when you begin, it is a good idea to rub them together to warm up first.

How do we know if we are rubbing correctly? Quite simply, because we feel better and more comfortable – almost straight away! Rubbing should induce a sense of calm and gentle warmth in the limb or body. The Taoists would probably call it 'a calm ecstasy'. So now, anyone can learn to merge the body with the infinite!

RUBBING THE STOMACH

Rubbing the stomach is likely to be the best place to begin. It can tackle general discomfort, heaviness, bloating, pain or cold sensations.

Make strokes mostly downwards; use the hands gently pressing, either over a single layer of clothing or the skin. Go slowly and gently, and stroke downward from the ribs – where you can feel the bones, to the bumps of the hip bones.

Make thirty-six strokes, using both hands together if you wish, firstly left of the navel, then centrally, then to the right of the navel. Gently move smoothly down the skin. Rest each time a short while, after each of the thirty-six strokes. If you get tired, try only nine slow strokes and then give it a rest.

Repeated regularly this will induce calm in the body. Try not to be anxious when performing this practice.

Keep a positive frame of mind and work steadily. The autonomic (self-regulatory) nervous system is some few million years old and used to healing, if we only give it a chance.

This exercise will calm the stomach, help sleep, warm the entire body and quieten the mind. It should also ease the breathing.

It can be performed sitting or standing, but is best done when lying in bed – where rubbing the stomach is sovereign in calming, settling the stomach and promoting sound sleep. Try a deep breath before you begin, letting the air gently stream out of the mouth.

Occasionally you may want to use further force and truly and firmly rub, press and deeply massage the whole lower abdomen. This can be especially warming and tonifying.

RUBBING THE ARMS

Rubbing the arms can also be performed at any time – usually it is done over your sleeves, but rubbing over bare skin is equally effective. Be careful not to press too hard. This rub can be easily done, stroking downwards from the shoulder joint, on the outside of the arm. When you have done this half a dozen times, gently turn the palm out, rotating the forearm, and stroke downwards along the inner surface, where it is softer.

You might finish by shaking the wrists, gently. And follow up by hanging down the forearm, letting all the weight drain out of it and loosely and slightly shaking the whole hand. This is excellent for Raynaud's syndrome, or persistent cold hands and feet.

RUBBING BEFORE SLEEP

The secret is to be one in mind and body – thoughts, bodily sensations and breath. Rubbing is an excellent aid to this. Dr Li Zhongzi said: 'When subduing the qi, there are three kinds of methods I use, conducive to sleep. There is the "sick dragon's sleep", where you breathe into the coiled-up knees; there is the "cold monkey's sleep", where you breathe into the knees, clutching them with the arms; and there is the "tortoise and crane sleep", where you breathe into the heels and knees.' Truly this saying is a treasure. To be warm and comfortable in your heels, knees and feet is vital for a good sleep. Try rubbing one sole, with the side of the foot, or big toe of the other. Rub the knees as well, and stroke down the thighs.

RUBBING THE KNEES

Rubbing the knees must be such a common thing to do! Who has not felt aches and pains in the knees? This exercise can be done anywhere and any time. Keep the hands and wrists loose – it is probably best to rub both knees at the same time. It is generally easier if you are sitting. But lying in bed is also good, drawing one or both knees up.

Try to maintain an even and circular motion with the palms. Hold the palm softly and gently.

This is *very* important. And the hands should be warm before you begin, as well. Try thirty-six circles one way and thirty-six the other. Finish up by stroking under and behind the knee; draw the hand up, pressing slightly into the hollow behind the knee. Take your time; relax into it.

RUBBING THE FEET

The Chinese make a big thing of rubbing the sole of the foot to lower blood-pressure; it is often mentioned in Qigong manuals. Sit upright and use the thumb or fingers to rub the sole of the foot, with gently regular movements. It can also be done in bed, as mentioned before, using the big toe of one foot to rub the sole of the other. It is most effective.

Appendix

Selections from Classical Texts

1. from the *Tao-Te Ching* (Way and its Power): the breath

> *The Spirit of the Valley will Never Die*
> *It may be named the Dark Female.*
> *The gateway to the Dark Female*
> *Is the root to all Heaven and Earth.*
> *Continuously one, as if always present,*
> *In use, it will never fail.*

Cultivation arises through a fertile valley. The spirit of the valley never dies because a valley is the proper place for life. Unlike us men, the women never live for themselves. The virtue of the Yin feminine, the 'dark female' lies in her 'detachment, resilience, ordinary chores, common and continuous usage'. This is also the role played by the breath. Nurture this spirit – and you will never confront death. Her gateway can be seen as the opening formed by the mouth and nose. The root to all Heaven and Earth – the channel for the breath – present in all life, passed back and forth.

In practice our breathing should be *continuously one*, fine and long. Gentle, it is 'as if always present', yet hardly sensed at all. It makes for contentment, relaxation and an unforced manner.

2. from the Taoist rhyme
A Mirror to the Medicine

> *the energy before we think*
> *the energy as we think,*
> *as we manage to get into it*
> *we always feel slightly tipsy!*
>
> *the days have moments they join*
> *the months have moments they join,*
> *delve into the still solid earth –*
> *settle expansion, extraction, wood and metal*
>
> *climb up the magpie bridge*
> *clamber down the magpie bridge,*
> *in heaven respond the stars*
> *on earth respond the tides*
>
> *their gentle breaths arise*
> *the receptive fire turns around,*
> *entering the calm Yellow Room*
> *we fashion the most precious jewels!*

This tract is at least a thousand years old. Find the time, position and place for your Qigong practice and the *fengshui* (wind–water) will be present. This is the 'moment they join'. Delve into the earth, there to read its stillness. Settle wood and metal, Yin and Yang, just the same. In Chinese legend the magpies form, one day a year, a bridge across the heavens so that the two lovers, the herdboy and spinning girl, can meet for the night. As their gentle breaths arise, the stars respond, and the tides beneath. Then the receptive fire of the body lights up the Yellow Room (yellow, the colour of the mean) and we enter, hand and hand together, the cave of jewels. Just remember *always natural in touching, always.*

3. from the Ming book (16th century)
Healing Without Medicines,
by Dr Li Zhongzi

THE MEDICINE OF THE MIND

The wisest doctors of ancient times could heal man's heart and innermost being. This was because they took the opportunity to act before a disease had begun. But what about present-day physicians? They only know how to heal someone already sick; they do not know how to heal a person's heart. It is a case of 'neglecting the root to chase after the branches'.

They do not enquire of the source of the trouble but boldly throw themselves into the stream of the disease. You may be looking for a speedy cure, but why do this!

They should recognize that disease originates in the heart, in our own innermost being. Calamities arise from our own actions. The fellow Buddha said:

> *It all lies in the constructs of the heart.*
> *The best is in never making false charges!*

It is for this reason that when strong emotions rise in the body, our true nature may be overturned in a twinkling. If this happens over a long time, eventually great sickness invades. And it is certainly not herbs or minerals which can cure this.

> *Doctors cannot enter the homes of criminals.*
> *Herbs cannot act where there is no love.*

In general, then, happiness acts the lord, while catastrophe plays the servant. Winkle out its mechanism and not one part will escape.

The cause of all this misery lies in the penalties of Heaven. It is the misery of 'self-destruct'. The penalties of Heaven originate from a former life where we accumulated too many transgressions. But while it is heaven and earth who dispatch us into this misery, our calamities find a source in our own heart.

Therefore while worldly thoughts and worries injure the heart, grief injures the lungs, resentment injures the liver, food and drink injure the spleen, and licentious desires injure the kidneys, the healing power of herbs are only half of it. The rest lies wholly beyond the strength of herbs. It must lie in the medicine of the mind.

What is meant by the 'medicine of the mind'? You might well listen to this poem I found in *Mirroring the Forest Temple*. It goes:

> *If your own mind is failing, your own mind will know it.*
> *The instant a thought comes make it a thought of healing.*
> *In general sickness is born and created in the mind.*
> *If the mind is kept safe, how can sickness arise?*

So it is essential to take control when casting out intrusion.

The ancient *Book of Medicine* has one phrase which instructs us all. It reads: 'Do not heal a disease which has already begun. Heal a disease which has not yet begun.' Treating a disease is not as good as treating where there is none; curing the body is not as good as curing the mind. By this I mean that curing others is simply not as good as first curing yourself!

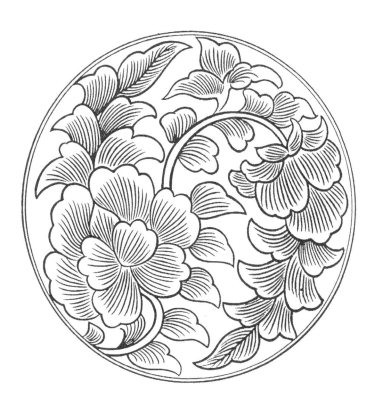

CPI Antony Rowe
Eastbourne, UK
September 02, 2024